Vegan Ba
Mouth-Wateri
Baking Recipes Including
Muffins, Breads, Cakes &
Cookies You Will Love!

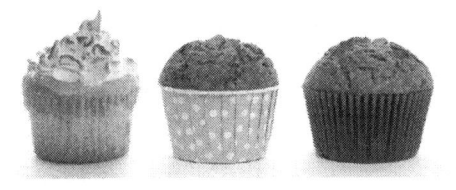

By Karen Greenvang (aka Karen Vegan)
Copyright ©Karen Greenvang 2016

www.HolisticWellnessBooks.com

All rights reserved. No part of this publication may be reproduced, stored in a retrieval system, or transmitted, in any form or by any means, electronic, mechanical, photocopying, recording or otherwise, without the prior written permission of the author and the publishers.

The scanning, uploading, and distribution of this book via the Internet, or via any other means, without the permission of the author is illegal and punishable by law. Please purchase only authorized electronic editions, and do not participate in or encourage electronic piracy of copyrighted materials.

All information in this book has been carefully researched and checked for factual accuracy. However, the author and publishers make no warranty, expressed or implied, that the information contained herein is appropriate for every individual, situation or purpose, and assume no responsibility for errors or omission. The reader assumes the risk and full responsibility for all actions, and the author will not be held liable for any loss or damage, whether consequential, incidental, and special or otherwise, that may result from the information presented in this publication.

All cooking is an experiment in a sense, and many people come to the same or similar recipe over time. All recipes in this book have been derived from author's personal experience. Should any bear a close resemblance to those used elsewhere, that is purely coincidental.

The book is not intended to provide medical advice or to take the place of medical advice and treatment from your personal physician. Readers are advised to consult their own doctors or other qualified health professionals regarding the treatment of medical conditions. The author shall not be held liable or responsible for any misunderstanding or misuse of the information contained in this book. The information is not intended to diagnose, treat or cure any disease.

It is important to remember that the author of this book is not a doctor/ medical professional. Only opinions based upon her own personal experiences or research are cited. THE AUTHOR DOES NOT OFFER MEDICAL ADVICE or prescribe any treatments. For any health or medical issues – you should be talking to your doctor first.

Vegan Baking

Vegan Baking-Introduction-5

Section I- Muffins-9

Section II- Breads-25

Section III-Cakes-39

Section IV-Cookies-55

Conclusion-65

More Books by Karen-67

Vegan Baking-Introduction

Countless studies have shown the health benefits of a vegan diet. Benefits such as sound nutrition, disease prevention, and overall physical health. A vegan way of life also has positive benefits on the environment, as modern commercial farming puts a lot of strain on the earth, both in terms of landmass and various greenhouse gases that have been proven to be a result of such farming methods.

A vegan approach to baking gives one the health benefits of whole grains, such as reduced risk of colon cancer. Fruits provide vitamins and minerals. Raw nuts and seeds are rich in heart-protecting Omega 3 fats, as well as healthy skin promoting properties.

This collection of recipes is free from highly refined carbohydrates, highly refined sugars and dairy. Raw, natural ingredients that are free from preservatives and additives, allow you to still enjoy baked treats while taking care of your body from within. The muffin recipes include a Rooibos tea infusion. Rooibos tea has become known world-wide for its anti-oxidant rich health benefits. It is also high in minerals and is known to promote healthy skin and hair. The anti-inflammatory properties of Rooibos help prevent heart related illnesses. It is also known to relieve hypertension, aid the digestive tract and help in the treatment of insomnia.

Cinnamon has been proven to possess many health benefits (including, anti-inflammatory properties). It reduces levels of total cholesterol, naturally controls blood sugar levels, helps fight against bacterial and fungal infections, and improves insulin sensitivity. Ginger is also known for its anti-inflammatory properties, as well as its ability to ease the discomfort of digestive issues, and is a great natural remedy for nausea and motion sickness. It also helps prevent muscle pain, and has cancer fighting properties.

The high fiber content of these recipes, not only promotes a healthy digestive system, but also gives them a low glycemic index, so they keep you full and satisfied for longer. This not only helps to further regulate blood sugar levels, but also keeps blood cholesterol at a healthy level.

The inclusion of healthy fats from a variety of raw seeds and nuts, and the use of both fresh and dried fruits, further make these recipes suitable to form the basis of healthy, energy sustaining, meals and snacks.

By substituting cow's milk for plant based options such as GMO-free soy, coconut and almond milk, as well as GMO-free soy yoghurt, further health benefits are provided. Soy milk is known to aid in the improvement of blood cholesterol, the prevention of certain cancers, and is a wonderful source of plant-based protein. Coconut milk is high in vitamins and minerals, as well as healthy unsaturated fats. Almond milk is known to help in weight management, contains no saturated fats, contributes to the healing process of muscles and promotes a healthy bone structure.

The use of raw brown sugar in some of the recipes, provides a less refined, healthier option to the highly refined white sugar that is generally used in baking. A nutritionally sound diet will always leave you with sustained energy, and all-round good health. A vegan diet is rich in plant based carbohydrates, proteins, vitamins and minerals, and will ensure that all your nutritional needs are met in the most natural way. When our diets are nutritionally sound, and satisfying, there is never any room for cravings for unhealthy, highly processed and refined options.

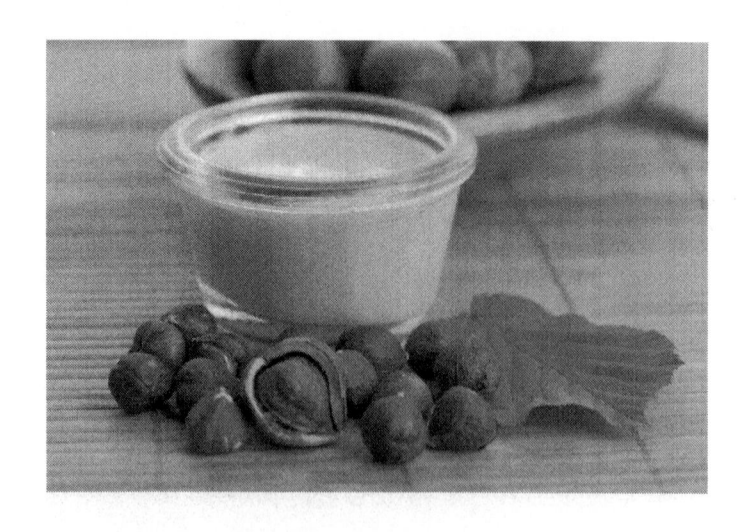

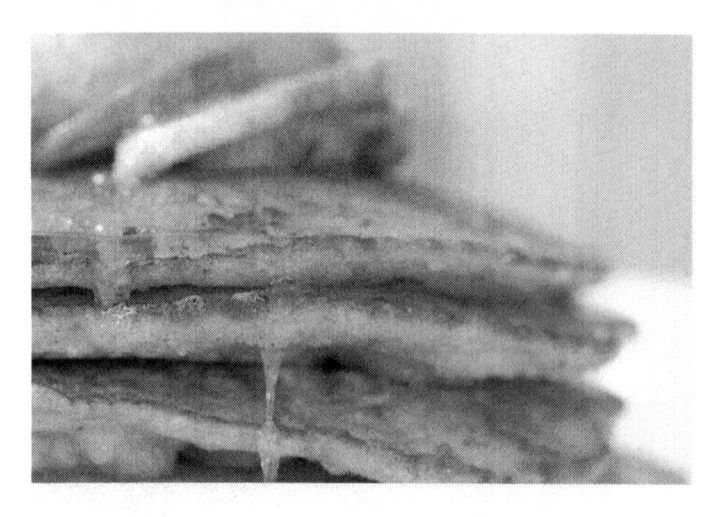

SECTION I
Muffins

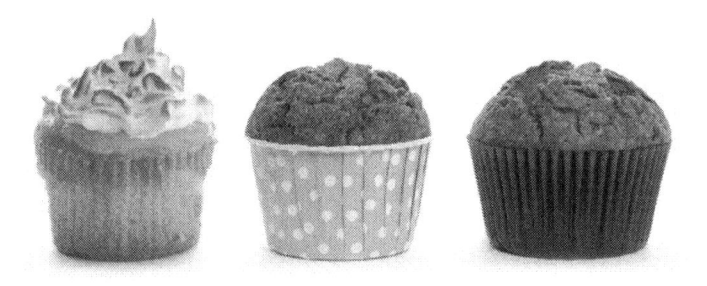

These muffin recipes are high in fiber, and full of energy sustaining carbohydrates. You will notice that these recipes do not use sugar, as the dried fruit, and grated apple provides a subtle hint of sweetness, making these muffins suitable as either a sweet snack when served with a natural fruit preserve, or as a more nutty, on-the-go snack when served with an organic nut butter of your choice. As with all the muffin recipes in this section, they are meant to be made as small, more cookie-sized muffins. This is because their high-fiber content deems them very filling. Also you can have two at a time without feeling like you have overdone it. One may also think that because these recipes do not include any fat or oil, other than the raw seeds or nuts, that they will be dry, but the high liquid content and the grated apple, which is a substitute for the more traditional binding agent of eggs, makes for very moist muffins. It is recommended that you don't peel the apple before grating it, as the fiber and vitamin C content of the apple rind adds further health benefits to the recipe. The basic recipe is the same for all variations, making it a very versatile basis for any additions that your personal tastes and creativity may desire.

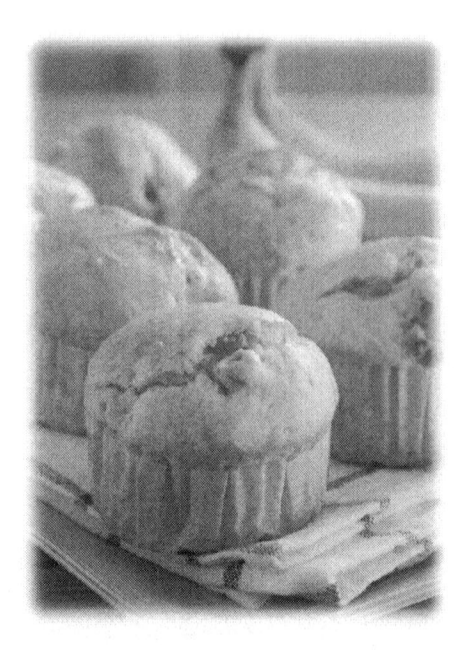

Rooibos Tea Infusion:

As mentioned in the introduction, these muffin recipes all include a Rooibos tea infusion as part of the wet ingredients. Either plain or fruit flavored Rooibos tea can be used. This infusion is made in a tea pot with an infusion basket and allowed to steep overnight.

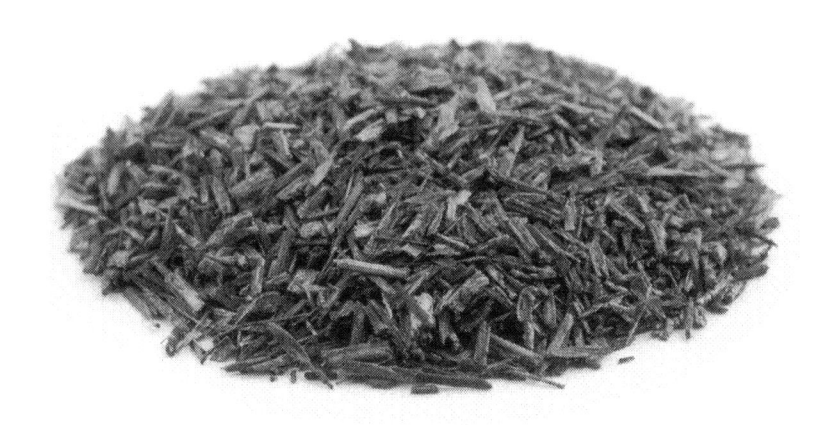

To make the Rooibos infusion:
1. Fill the infusion basket of your teapot half way, with organic cinnamon sticks or bark.
2. Place two Rooibos tea bags on top of the cinnamon. If you are using loose tea leaves, you will need approximately four teaspoons (20ml) of the leaves.
3. Fill the pot with boiling water, and allow to steep overnight.

This infusion is also delicious, and incredibly healthy to drink either cold or hot. Drinking it cold is refreshing, while drinking it hot is comforting. When drinking it hot, the addition of coconut, or almond milk will complement the strong cinnamon flavor.

This infusion can also be used instead of plain water when cooking oatmeal. It will add a delicious flavor, and extra health benefits to your average bowl of oatmeal. Again, the addition of coconut, or almond milk will complement the strong cinnamon flavor.

This really is a very versatile infusion, with all the added health benefits of the Rooibos tea and cinnamon.

Basic Bran Muffins

Preheat the oven to 390 degrees (200 degrees Celsius). And grease two non-stick small muffin trays with coconut oil or vegan friendly cooking spray. Makes 30 cookie-sized muffins.

Dry ingredients:

- 1 ¼ Cups (310ml) Organic whole wheat flour
- ¼ cup (60ml) Organic wheat bran
- 2 teaspoons (10ml) baking soda
- 2 teaspoons (10ml) baking powder
- 1 teaspoon (5ml) ground cinnamon
- ½ Cup (125ml) seed mix (this can include pumpkin, sesame, flax seeds)
- ¼ Cup (60ml) Raisins, dried mixed berries, or chopped dates. This is to your choice.

Wet Ingredients:

- 1 Cup (250ml) soy, almond or coconut milk
- 1 ½ Cups (375ml) Rooibos tea infusion
- ½ Cup (125ml) Soy yoghurt
- 1 medium sized apple, cored and grated
- 1 Tablespoon (15ml) vanilla essence or vanilla extract

Instructions:

1. In a large mixing bowl, combine all the dry ingredients.
2. Combine the wet ingredients together in a large measuring jug and add to the dry ingredients.
3. Mix well, making sure to incorporate lots of air into the mixture.
4. Fill each muffin cup with two tablespoons (30ml) of the batter. Because the recipe includes both baking soda, and baking powder, they will rise sufficiently.
5. Bake for 25 minutes.
6. Once baked, allow the muffins to cool in the tins for approximately ten minutes before turning out onto a wire rack to cool.

Banana Muffins

Preheat the oven to 390 degrees (200 degrees Celsius). And grease two non-stick small muffin trays with coconut oil or vegan friendly cooking spray. Makes 30 cookie-sized muffins.

Dry ingredients:

- 1 ¼ Cups (310ml) Organic whole wheat flour
- ¼ Cup(60ml) Organic wheat bran
- 2 teaspoons (10ml) baking soda
- 2 teaspoons (10ml) baking powder
- 1 teaspoon (5ml) ground cinnamon
- ½ Cup (125ml) seed mix (this can included pumpkin, sesame, flax seeds)
- ¼ Cup (60ml) Raisins, dried mixed berries, or chopped dates. This is to your choice.

Wet Ingredients:

- 1 Cup (250ml) soy, almond or coconut milk
- 1 ½ Cups (375ml) Rooibos tea infusion
- ½ Cup (125ml) Soy yoghurt
- 1 medium sized apple, cored and grated.
- 1 Tablespoon (15ml) vanilla essence or vanilla extract
- 3 medium sized, very ripe bananas, mashed.

Instructions:

1. In a large mixing bowl, combine all the dry ingredients.
2. Combine the wet ingredients together in a large measuring jug and add to the dry ingredients.
3. Mix well, making sure to incorporate lots of air into the mixture. Fill each muffin cup with two tablespoons (30ml) of the batter. Because the recipe includes both baking soda, and baking powder, they will rise sufficiently.
4. Bake for 25 minutes.
5. Once baked, allow the muffins to cool in the tins for approximately ten minutes before turning out onto a wire rack to cool.

Orange Ginger Poppy Seed Muffins

Preheat the oven to 390 degrees (200 degrees Celsius). And grease two non-stick small muffin trays with coconut oil or vegan friendly cooking spray. Makes 30 cookie-sized muffins.

Dry ingredients:

- 1 ¼ (310ml) Cups Organic whole wheat flour
- ¼ Cup (60ml) Organic wheat bran
- 2 teaspoons (10ml) baking soda
- 2 teaspoons (10ml) baking powder
- 1 teaspoon (5ml) ground cinnamon
- 1 teaspoon (5ml) of freshly grated ginger root
- ½ Cup (125ml) poppy seeds

Wet Ingredients:

- 1 Cup (250ml) soy, almond or coconut milk
- 1 ½ Cups (375ml) Rooibos tea infusion
- ½ Cup (125ml) Soy yoghurt
- 1 medium sized apple, cored and grated
- 1 Tablespoon (15ml) vanilla essence or vanilla extract
- 1 Medium-sized orange, rind grated and flesh cut into pieces.

Instructions:

1. In a large mixing bowl, combine all the dry ingredients.
2. Combine the wet ingredients together in a large measuring jug and add to the dry ingredients.
3. Mix well, making sure to incorporate lots of air into the mixture. Fill each muffin cup with two tablespoons (30ml) of the batter. Because the recipe includes both baking soda, and baking powder, they will rise sufficiently.
4. Bake for 25 minutes.
5. Once baked, allow the muffins to cool in the tins for approximately ten minutes before turning out onto a wire rack to cool.

Lemon Poppy Seed Muffins

Preheat the oven to 390 degrees (200 degrees Celsius). And grease two non-stick small muffin trays with coconut oil or vegan friendly cooking spray. Makes 30 cookie-sized muffins.

Dry ingredients:

- 1 ¼ Cups (310ml) Organic whole wheat flour
- ¼ Cup (60ml) Organic wheat bran
- 2 teaspoons (10ml) baking soda
- 2 teaspoons (10ml) baking powder
- 1 teaspoon (5ml) ground cinnamon
- 1 teaspoon (5ml) of freshly grated ginger root
- ½ Cup (125ml) poppy seeds

Wet Ingredients:

- 1 Cup(250ml) soy, almond or coconut milk
- 1 ½ Cups (375ml) Rooibos tea infusion
- ½ Cup (125ml) Soy yoghurt
- 1 medium sized apple, cored and grated
- 1 Tablespoon (15ml) vanilla essence or vanilla extract
- 1 Medium-sized lemon, rind grated and flesh cut into pieces.

Instructions:

1. In a large mixing bowl, combine all the dry ingredients.
2. Combine the wet ingredients together in a large measuring jug and add to the dry ingredients.
3. Mix well, making sure to incorporate lots of air into the mixture. Fill each muffin cup with two tablespoons (30ml) of the batter. Because the recipe includes both baking soda, and baking powder, they will rise sufficiently.
4. Bake for 25 minutes.
5. Once baked, allow the muffins to cool in the tins for approximately ten minutes before turning out onto a wire rack to cool.

Apple Chia Muffins

Preheat the oven to 390 degrees (200 degrees Celsius). And grease two non-stick small muffin trays with coconut oil or vegan friendly cooking spray. Makes 30 cookie-sized muffins.

Dry ingredients:

- 1 ¼ Cups (310ml) Organic whole wheat flour
- ¼ Cup (60ml) Organic wheat bran
- 2 teaspoons (10ml) baking soda
- 2 teaspoons (10ml) baking powder
- 1 teaspoon (10ml) ground cinnamon
- 1 teaspoon (10ml) of freshly grated ginger root
- ¼ Cup (60ml) Raisins, chopped dates or dried mixed berries, to your choice.
- ½ Cup (125ml) Chia seeds

Wet Ingredients:

- 1 Cup (250ml) soy, almond or coconut milk
- 1 ½ Cups (375ml) Rooibos tea infusion
- ½ Cup (125ml) Soy yoghurt
- 1 medium sized apple, cored and grated
- 1 Tablespoon (15ml) vanilla essence or vanilla extract

Instructions:

1. In a large mixing bowl, combine all the dry ingredients.
2. Combine the wet ingredients together in a large measuring jug and add to the dry ingredients.
3. Mix well, making sure to incorporate lots of air into the mixture. Fill each muffin cup with two tablespoons (30ml) of the batter. Because the recipe includes both baking soda, and baking powder, they will rise sufficiently.
4. Bake for 25 minutes.
5. Once baked, allow the muffins to cool in the tins for approximately ten minutes before turning out onto a wire rack to cool.

Carrot Bran Muffins

Preheat the oven to 390 degrees (200 degrees Celsius). And grease two non-stick small muffin trays with coconut oil or vegan friendly cooking spray. Makes 30 cookie-sized muffins.

Dry ingredients:

- 1 ¼ (310ml) Cups Organic whole wheat flour
- ¼ Cup (60ml) Organic wheat bran
- 2 teaspoons (10ml) baking soda
- 2 teaspoons (10ml) baking powder
- 1 teaspoon (5ml) ground cinnamon
- 1 teaspoon (5ml) of freshly grated ginger root
- ¼ Cup (60ml) sultanas
- 1 Tablespoon (15ml) Desiccated Coconut
- 1 Tablespoon (15ml) chopped Pecan Nuts

Wet Ingredients:

- 1 Cup (250ml) soy, almond or coconut milk
- 1 ½ Cups (375ml) Rooibos tea infusion
- ½ Cup (125ml) Soy yoghurt
- 1 medium sized apple, cored and grated
- 1 medium sized carrot, grated
- 1 Tablespoon (15ml) vanilla essence or vanilla extract

Instructions:

1. In a large mixing bowl, combine all the dry ingredients.
2. Combine the wet ingredients together in a large measuring jug and add to the dry ingredients.
3. Mix well, making sure to incorporate lots of air into the mixture. Fill each muffin cup with two tablespoons (30ml) of the batter.
4. Bake for 25 minutes.
5. Once baked, allow the muffins to cool in the tins for ten minutes before turning out onto a wire rack to cool.

SECTION II

Breads

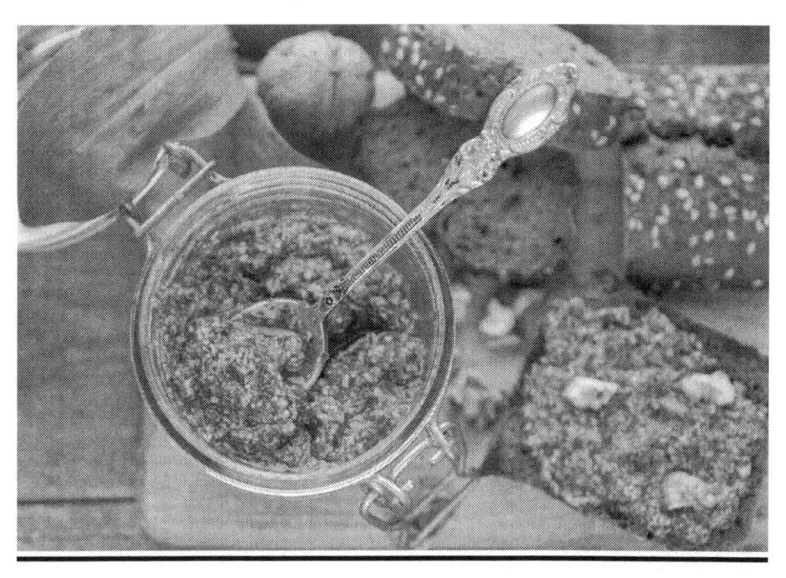

Modern day commercial baking has led to a generation that has only ever known the highly refined, stodgy breads that are available on supermarket shelves. These breads have little health benefits, are packed with preservatives, and their quick energy releasing nature can play havoc with blood sugar levels. As a result, bread has come to take a really bad wrap over the last few decades. But, including bread in your diet does not have to be detrimental to your health or weight management goals.

By choosing to bake your own bread you are taking control of your health on another level. You are taking out the commercial additives and preservatives, and going back to basics.

The breads in this section are all made with wholegrain organic flours, and are simple and easy to make. Whole grains help to sustain energy for longer, and their high fiber content is incredibly helpful to the digestive system.

The inclusion of healthy fats in the form of raw seeds and nuts, adds that extra health boost. Not to mention the high content of vitamins and minerals found in the raw nuts and seeds. With the use of Tahini, which is sesame seed paste, well known to Middle Eastern cooking, the heart-healthy fat content is increased.

By now we all know about the added health benefits of including fruit in our diets. Fruits are high in vitamins, minerals and dietary fiber, and add a little sweetness to the health bread variations.

Once you try these breads, you will see how there is no reason why bread should be labelled "unhealthy". Furthermore, the meditative benefits that come from kneading your own bread, along with the comforting smell of it baking, will make you wonder why you never made your own bread before.

Whole Wheat Seeded Health Bread

This basic recipe forms the canvas on which the rest of the health bread recipes in this book are formed. This recipe is incredibly versatile, and makes a delicious, moist health bread that can be enjoyed with any kind of meal. It is also delicious served with natural fruit preserves and organic, natural nut butters. These health breads don't require kneading, as the ingredients form more of a batter than a dough once mixed together.

Preheat the oven 390 degrees (200 degrees Celsius).

This recipe **yields three loaves**, so you will need to grease three medium-sized loaf tins, very well, with either coconut oil or vegan friendly cooking spray.

Ingredients:
- 4 Cups (1kg) Organic Whole Wheat Flour
- ½ Cup (125ml) Organic Raw Brown Sugar
- 1 Tablespoon (15ml) Organic Sea Salt
- 2 Tablespoons (30ml) Instant Dry yeast
- ¼ Cup (60ml) Seed mix (can include pumpkin,

sesame, flax seeds)
- ¼ Cup (60ml) Poppy Seeds
- 4 Cups (1litre) Lukewarm Water.

Instructions:

1. Dissolve the sugar in the lukewarm water and sprinkle the yeast over the top.
2. Cover tightly with cling film and a dish towel, and set aside for the yeast to activate, it will start to bubble when it has activated.
3. In a large mixing bowl, mix together the flour, seeds and salt,
4. Add the water, sugar and yeast mixture and mix very well to form a slightly runny batter.
5. Divide the batter equally amongst the loaf tins.
6. Cover them with cling film and set aside in a warm place until the batter has risen and the loaves have doubled in size.
7. Bake for 45-50 minutes, until a dark crust has formed and the bread sounds hollow when tapped.
8. You can also check that they are completely baked by using skewer.
9. Allow the loaves to cool in the tins for ten minutes before turning out onto a cooling rack.

Spicy, Fruity Whole Wheat Health Bread

The addition of fruit and baking spices to this variation makes this bread a really healthy tea-time treat when topped with natural fruit preserves and/or organic, natural nut butters. It also makes a great addition to any breakfast, and serves as a wonderful accompaniment to your favorite lunch time salad.

Preheat the oven 390 degrees (200 degrees Celsius).

This recipe **yields three loaves**, so you will need to grease three medium-sized loaf tins, very well, with either coconut oil or vegan friendly cooking spray.

Ingredients:

- 4 Cups (1kg) Organic Whole Wheat Flour
- ½ Cup (125ml) Organic Raw Brown Sugar
- 1 Tablespoon (15ml) Organic Sea Salt
- 2 Tablespoons (30ml) Instant Dry yeast
- ¼ Cup (60ml) Seed mix (can included pumpkin, sesame, flax seeds)
- ¼ Cup (60ml) Poppy Seeds
- 1 medium-sized apple, cored and grated (include

the peel to add extra fiber and flavor)
- ¼ Cup (60ml) Raisins, or dried berry mix.
- 1 teaspoon (5ml) Ground Cinnamon
- 1 teaspoon (5ml) Ground Baking Spice Mix.
- 4 Cups (1 litre) Lukewarm Water.

Instructions:

1. Dissolve the sugar in the lukewarm water and sprinkle the yeast over the top.
2. Cover tightly with cling film and a dish towel and set aside for the yeast to activate, it will start to bubble when it has activated. In a large mixing bowl, mix together the flour, seeds, fruits, spices and salt.
3. Add the water, sugar and yeast mixture and mix very well to form a slightly runny batter.
4. Divide the batter equally amongst the loaf tins.
5. Cover them with cling film and set aside in a warm place until the batter has risen and the loaves have doubled in size.
6. Bake for 45-50 minutes, until a dark crust has formed and the bread sounds hollow when tapped.
7. You can also check that they are completely baked by using skewer. Allow the loaves to cool in the tins for ten minutes before turning out onto a cooling rack.

Date, Pecan and Bran Whole Wheat Health Bread

The inclusion of wheat bran, dates and pecan nuts to this variation give it a nutty flavor, and an added fiber kick from the wheat bran and the dates. This recipe also includes cinnamon to add a little comfort to compliment the nutty flavor. As with the other health breads in this section, this variation can be enjoyed with almost any meal, and also goes very well topped with natural fruit preserves and organic nut butters.

Preheat the oven 390 degrees (200 degrees Celsius).

This recipe **yields three loaves**, so you will need to grease three medium-sized loaf tins, very well, with either coconut oil or vegan friendly cooking spray.

Ingredients:

- 3 ½ Cups (875ml) Organic Whole Wheat Flour
- ½ Cup (125ml) Wheat Bran
- ½ Cup (125ml) Organic Raw Brown Sugar
- 1 Tablespoon (15ml) Organic Sea Salt
- 2 Tablespoons (30ml) Instant Dry yeast

- ¼ Cup (60ml) Raw Pecan nuts, chopped
- ¼ Cup (60ml) Chopped Dates
- 1 teaspoon (5ml) Ground Cinnamon
- 4 Cups (1litre) Lukewarm Water.

Instructions:

1. Dissolve the sugar in the lukewarm water and sprinkle the yeast over the top.
2. Cover tightly with cling film and a dish towel and set aside for the yeast to activate, it will start to bubble when it has activated.
3. In a large mixing bowl, mix together the flour, seeds, fruits, spices and salt.
4. Add the water, sugar and yeast mixture and mix very well to form a slightly runny batter.
5. Divide the batter equally amongst the loaf tins.
6. Cover them with cling film and set aside in a warm place until the batter has risen and the loaves have doubled in size.
7. Bake for 45-50 minutes, until a dark crust has formed and the bread sounds hollow when tapped.
8. You can also check that they are completely baked by using a skewer.
9. Allow the loaves to cool in the tins for ten minutes before turning out onto a cooling rack.

Wholegrain Rye Bread

There is a vast amount of research into the health benefits, and blood sugar controlling properties of rye flour. Rye flour is known to form the basis of traditional German breads, and provides a wholesome, fiber-rich option to bread baking. By including whole wheat flour in this recipe, the fiber content is further increased. Rye has a very distinct flavor that is complimented by the addition of caraway seeds, making this bread a very satisfying side to any savory meal. The inclusion of Tahini, sesame paste, adds to the flavor of this bread, while giving you the benefits of its heart-healthy omega fat content. It can, however also be enjoyed with sweeter topping options. Making this bread has the added benefit of meditation while kneading the dough.

Preheat the oven 390 degrees (200 degrees Celsius).

This recipe **yields three loaves**, so you will need to grease three medium-sized loaf tins, very well, with either coconut oil or vegan friendly cooking spray.

Ingredients:

- 2 Cups (500mls) Organic Pure Rye Flour
- 2 Cups (500mls Organic Whole Wheat Flour
- 1 Tablespoon (15ml) Organic Sea Salt
- 2 Tablespoons (30ml) Caraway Seeds
- 1 Tablespoon (15ml) Dry Instant yeast
- 3 Cups (750ml) Lukewarm water
- 2 Tablespoons (30ml) Organic Raw Brown Sugar

Instructions:

1. Dissolve the sugar in the lukewarm water and sprinkle the yeast over the top.
2. Cover tightly with cling film and a dish towel, set aside until the yeast has activated.
3. Sift the rye, whole wheat flours and salt together into a large mixing bowl.
4. Add the caraway seeds and rub-in the Tahini paste.
5. Once the yeast has activated, add the water and mix all together to form a workable dough.
6. Turn the dough out onto a lightly floured surface and knead for about 10 to 15 minutes, until the dough has stopped sticking to your hands, and is smooth and elastic.
7. Place the dough back into the mixing bowl, cover with cling film and a warm, damp dish towel.
8. Set aside for about an hour until the dough has

doubled in size. Punch the dough down to release a little of the air, and divide equally amongst the three loaf tins.
9. Cover the loaves with cling film and a warm damp dish cloth, and set aside until the loaves have doubled in size.
10. Bake for 35 minutes, or until a skewer comes out clean and the loaves sound hollow when tapped.
11. Allow to cool for 10 minutes in the tins before turning out onto a cooling rack.

Whole Wheat Rye Bagels

The traditional deli bagel can be very heavy, since it is made with highly refined white flour. These bagels pack a high fiber punch and the inclusion of Tahini paste adds a little healthy fat. The addition of rye flour adds to the flavor, making these bagels a light, healthy, hearty alternative to your regular heavy white bagel. By boiling the bagels before baking them, they still have that familiar bagel texture and golden brown finish. As with all the breads in this book, these bagels go well with any meal, and make a great start to that perfect lunch time, or snack time, sandwich. Makes 26-28 bagels.

Preheat the oven 390 degrees (200 degrees Celsius).

Ingredients:

- 2 Cups (500mls) Organic Pure Rye Flour
- 2 Cups (500mls) Organic Whole Wheat Flour
- 1 Tablespoon (15ml) Organic Sea Salt
- 1 Tablespoon (15ml) Dry Instant yeast
- 3 Cups (750ml) Lukewarm water
- 2 Tablespoons (30ml) Organic Raw Brown Sugar

Instructions:

1. Dissolve the sugar in the lukewarm water and sprinkle the yeast over the top.
2. Cover tightly with cling film and a dish towel, set aside until the yeast has activated.
3. Sift the rye, whole wheat flours and salt together in a large mixing bowl.
4. Rub-in the Tahini paste.
5. Once the yeast has activated, add the water and mix all together to form a workable dough.
6. Turn the dough out onto a lightly floured surface and knead for about 10 to 15 minutes, until the dough has stopped sticking to your hands, and is smooth and elastic.
7. Place the dough back into the mixing bowl, cover with cling film and a warm damp dish towel.
8. Set aside for about an hour until the dough has doubled in size. Using a ¼ Cup (60ml) measuring cup, measure out ¼ cup-sized (60ml) balls of the dough.
9. Roll each ball into a rope shape before forming into a loop to make the bagel shape.
10. Once all the dough has been made into bagels, set them aside on a lightly floured surface, and cover with cling film.
11. Give about 45 minutes, until they have doubled in

size.
12. Fill a heavy-based saucepan with water, and bring it to the boil. Boil each bagel for 1 minute, turning it over at the 30 second mark. Place the bagels on non-stick baking trays, you might want to give them a light spray with vegan friendly cooking spray, and bake for 25 minutes, or until golden brown.
13. Allow to cool for 10 minutes on the trays before turning out onto a cooling rack.

SECTION III

Cakes

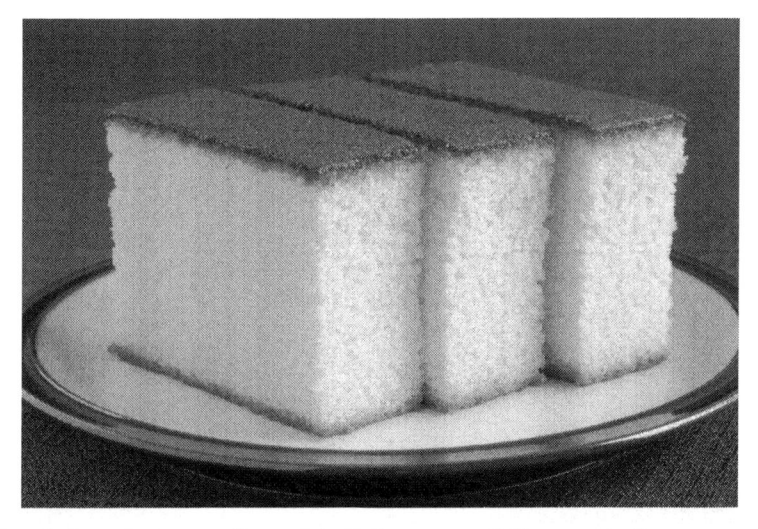

Special celebrations such as birthdays, weddings, and any kind of party, just aren't complete without cake. That slice of cake is what we all look forward to when we plan a party, it's a real treat.

These recipes prove that you can have your cake and eat it, without any guilt. By using organic, preservative free flours you are omitting all the additives that come with commercially baked cakes. The use of healthy fat options, such as coconut oil, raw nuts and seeds, and desiccated coconut, replaces the normally high saturated fat content of bakery cakes with unsaturated, heart-healthy fats.

The addition of fruit to some of these recipes adds extra vitamins and minerals to every slice.

The light frosting options are a great alternative to the heavy, rich frostings that are common on commercially baked cakes, and by using natural, raw ingredients, they are also a healthier frosting option.

Basic Sponge Cake

This recipe forms the basis for the sponge cake recipes that follow, making it versatile and easy to adapt to any occasion. The simple frosting adds the extra benefit of vitamin C from the orange juice, and orange rind is high in flavonoids and phytonutrients, as well as fiber, it also has great immune boosting qualities.

Serves: 12

Preheat the oven to 390 degrees (200 degrees Celsius).

Grease a round cake tin with coconut oil, or vegan friendly cooking spray.

Ingredients:

- ¼ Cup (60ml) Coconut Oil
- 1 ½ Cups (375ml) Organic cake flour
- ¾ Cup (200ml) Organic white sugar
- 2 teaspoons (10ml) Baking Powder
- ½ Cup (125ml) Soy or Almond milk
- ½ Cup (125ml) Soy yoghurt
- 1 teaspoon (10ml) Vanilla essence.

Instructions:

1. In an electric mixer beat the coconut oil at a high

speed until it is light and fluffy.
2. Add the sugar and return to high speed, beat until all the sugar has dissolved.
3. In a separate bowl, sift the flour and baking powder together.
4. Combine the soy or almond milk and soy yoghurt in a jug, and add the vanilla.
5. With your electric mixer on a slow speed, slowly add the soy or almond milk and yoghurt mixture to the coconut oil and sugar mix, and mix well.
6. Keeping the electric mixer at a slow speed, slowly add the flour and baking powder mixture.
7. Once all is combined, turn up the speed for a few minutes to incorporate as much air into the mixture as possible, this will help make the sponge light and fluffy.
8. Pour the cake batter into the baking tin and bake for about one hour, or until a skewer comes out clean.
9. Leave to cool in the tin for ten minutes before turning out onto a cooling rack.

For the Frosting:

- 1cup (250ml) Organic fresh orange juice (you can squeeze this yourself)
- ½ Cup (125ml) Frosting sugar, (this is powdery in

texture), sifted.
- 1 Tablespoon (15ml) Orange rind

Instructions:

1. It's best to make this frosting just before you pour it over the cake. Combine the orange juice and sugar and mix well to form a thick, paste, it should have the consistency of yoghurt, so not too runny, but still pourable.
2. Once the cake has completely cooled pour the frosting over it and sprinkle with the orange rind.
3. Allow the frosting to set before serving.

Chocolate Sponge Cake

Who can resist a slice of chocolate cake? This recipe makes a rich and chocolatey cake with all the added health benefits of raw cocoa. Raw cocoa provides you with a dose of essential minerals such as magnesium, calcium, sulphur, zinc, iron, manganese and potassium. Raw cocoa has also become known for its high anti-oxidant benefits, as well as its ability to aid in the lowering of blood pressure. So there really is no reason why not to have a slice of this chocolate cake.

The frosting is made with coconut oil and almond milk, so it adds an extra dose of heart-healthy fats and essential minerals, as do the raw almonds that form the topping.

Serves: 12

Preheat the oven to 390 degrees (200 degrees Celsius).

Grease a round cake tin with coconut oil, or vegan friendly cooking spray.

Ingredients:
- ¼ Cup (60ml) Coconut Oil
- 1 ½ Cups (375ml) Organic cake flour

- ¼ Cup (60ml) Raw organic cocoa powder
- ¾ Cup (200ml) Organic white sugar
- 2 teaspoons (10ml) Baking Powder
- ½ Cup (125ml) Soy or Almond milk
- ½ Cup (125ml) Soy yoghurt
- 1 teaspoon (10ml) Vanilla essence.

Instructions:

1. In an electric mixer beat the coconut oil at a high speed until it is light and fluffy, add the sugar and return to high speed, beat until all the sugar has dissolved.
2. In a separate bowl, sift the flour, cocoa powder and baking powder together.
3. Combine the soy or almond milk and soy yoghurt in a jug, and add the vanilla.
4. With your electric mixer on a slow speed, slowly add the soy or almond milk and yoghurt mixture to the coconut oil and sugar mixture, and mix well.
5. Keeping the electric mixer at a slow speed, slowly add the flour, baking powder, and cocoa powder mixture.
6. Once all is combined, turn up the speed for a few minutes to incorporate as much air into the mixture as possible, this will help make the sponge light and fluffy.

7. Pour the cake batter into the baking tin and bake for about one hour, or until a skewer comes out clean.
8. Leave to cool in the tin for ten minutes before turning out onto a cooling rack.

For the frosting

- ¼ Cup (60ml) coconut oil
- 2 Cups (500ml) Frosting sugar, (this is powdery in texture)
- ¼ Cup (60ml) Almond milk
- 2 Tablespoons (30ml) Raw organic cocoa powder
- 1 Teaspoon (5ml) Vanilla Essence
- 2 Tablespoons (30) Raw almonds, chopped.

Instructions:

1. Sift the powdered icing sugar and raw cocoa together into a mixing bowl.
2. In an electric mixer, beat the coconut oil at a very high speed until it becomes smooth and creamy.
3. Reduce the speed and slowly add the sugar and cocoa powder mixture and combine well.
4. Keeping the electric mixer at a slow speed, add the almond milk and vanilla essence.
5. Turn up the speed and mix until you have a light, fluffy frosting.

6. Once the cake has completely cooled, cover it generously with the frosting and sprinkle with the chopped almonds.
7. This cake goes very well served with freshly brewed organic coffee.

Orange Ginger Sponge Cake

Ginger is known for its anti-inflammatory properties, as well as its ability to ease the discomfort of digestive issues. It is known to help prevent muscle pain, and cancer. Orange rind is high in flavonoids and phytonutrients, as well as fiber, and has great immune boosting qualities. The hint of spices and cinnamon adds a comforting flavor to this recipe. The simple orange juice frosting as used with the basic sponge cake goes best with this variation, and adds an extra vitamin C boost.

Serves: 12

Preheat the oven to 390 degrees (200 degrees Celsius).

Grease a round cake tin with coconut oil, or vegan friendly cooking spray.

Ingredients:

- ¼ Cup (60ml) Coconut Oil
- 1 ½ Cups (375ml) Organic cake flour
- ¾ Cup (200ml) Organic white sugar
- 2 teaspoons (10ml) Baking Powder
- 2 Tablespoons (30ml) Freshly grated ginger root
- 1 teaspoon (5ml) Ground Cinnamon
- 1 teaspoon (5ml) Baking spice mix

- ½ Cup (125ml) Soy or Almond milk
- ½ Cup (125ml) Soy yoghurt
- 1 teaspoon (10ml) Vanilla essence.

Instructions:

1. In an electric mixer beat the coconut oil at a high speed until it is light and fluffy, add the sugar and return to high speed, beat until all the sugar has dissolved.
2. In a separate bowl, sift the flour, baking powder, and spices together, add the orange rind.
3. Combine the soy or almond milk and soy yoghurt in a jug, and add the vanilla. With your electric mixer on a slow speed, slowly add the soy or almond milk and yoghurt mixture to the coconut oil and sugar mix, and mix well.
4. Keeping the electric mixer at a slow speed, slowly add the dry ingredients.
5. Once all is combined, turn up the speed for a few minutes to incorporate as much air into the mixture as possible, this will help make the sponge light and fluffy.
6. Pour the cake batter into the baking tin and bake for about one hour, or until a skewer comes out clean.
7. Leave to cool in the tin for ten minutes before

turning out onto a cooling rack.

For the Frosting:

- 1cup (250ml) Organic fresh orange juice (you can squeeze this yourself)
- ½ Cup (125ml) Frosting sugar, (this is powdery in texture), sifted.
- 1 Tablespoon (15ml) Orange rind

Instructions:

1. It's best to make this frosting just before you pour it over the cake. Combine the orange juice and sugar and mix well to form a thick, paste, it should have the consistency of yoghurt, so not too runny, but still pourable.
2. Once the cake has completely cooled pour the frosting over it and sprinkle with the orange rind.
3. Allow the frosting to set before serving.

Whole Wheat Carrot and Pineapple Cake

This cake is so wholesome that it could be a meal on its own! Packed with fiber, vitamins, minerals and healthy fats, it's so nutritious that you won't believe you are actually eating cake! The carrots provide a good dose of vitamin A, while the pineapple and sultanas add the vitamin C, manganese and a whack of anti-oxidants. The addition of raw pecan nuts gives an extra boost of magnesium, zinc and potassium. Pecan nuts are also known to help lower bad cholesterol. The desiccated coconut not only adds a little extra heart-healthy unsaturated fats, but also compliments the flavor of the pineapple and spices. By using whole wheat flour, instead of the usual cake flour, the fiber content is further boosted. The lemony twist that is added by the light frosting adds some more vitamin C, as well as a complimenting zing to the overall taste your slice.

Serves: 12

Preheat the oven to 390 degrees (200 degrees Celsius).

Grease a large round cake tin with coconut oil, or vegan friendly cooking spray.

Ingredients:

- 2 ½ Cups (625ml) Whole Wheat Flour
- 2 teaspoons (10ml) Baking Powder
- 2 teaspoons (10ml) Baking Soda
- 1 teaspoon (5ml) Ground Cinnamon
- 1 teaspoon (5ml) Baking spice mix
- 1 teaspoon (5ml) Freshly grated ginger root
- 1 tablespoon (15ml) Desiccated coconut
- 1 ½ Cups (375ml) Raw brown sugar
- 1 ½ Cups (375ml) Coconut Oil
- 2 Cups (500ml) Grated fresh carrot
- 1 Cup (250ml) Crushed pineapple (this can be the tinned variety)
- ½ Cup (125ml) Raw Pecan nuts, chopped
- ½ Cup (125ml) Golden Sultanas.

Instructions:

1. In a large mixing bowl combine the whole wheat flour, baking powder, baking soda, cinnamon, spice mix, fresh ginger, chopped pecan nuts, sultanas and desiccated coconut.
2. Using an electric mixer beat the coconut oil and sugar together on a high speed until light and fluffy, and all the sugar had dissolved.
3. Turn the speed down to a low pulse and add the grated carrot and crushed pineapple, mix well.

4. Slowly spoon in the dry ingredients, while keeping the electric mixer going at a slow speed.
5. Once all the ingredients are combined, turn the electric mixer up to a medium speed and mix well for about five minutes, making sure to incorporate as much air into the mixture as possible.
6. Pour the mixture into the cake tin and bake for one hour, or until a skewer comes out clean.
7. Allow to cool in the tin for ten minutes before turning out onto a cooling rack.

For the Frosting:

- 1 Cup (250ml) Organic fresh lemon juice (you can squeeze this yourself)
- ½ Cup (125ml) Frosting sugar, (this is powdery in texture), sifted.
- 1 Tablespoon (15ml) Lemon rind

Instructions:

1. It's best to make this frosting just before you pour it over the cake. Combine the orange juice and sugar and mix well to form a thick, paste, it should have the consistency of yoghurt, so not too runny, but still pourable.
2. Once the cake has completely cooled pour the frosting over it and sprinkle with the lemon rind.

3. Allow the frosting to set before serving.

SECTION IV
Cookies

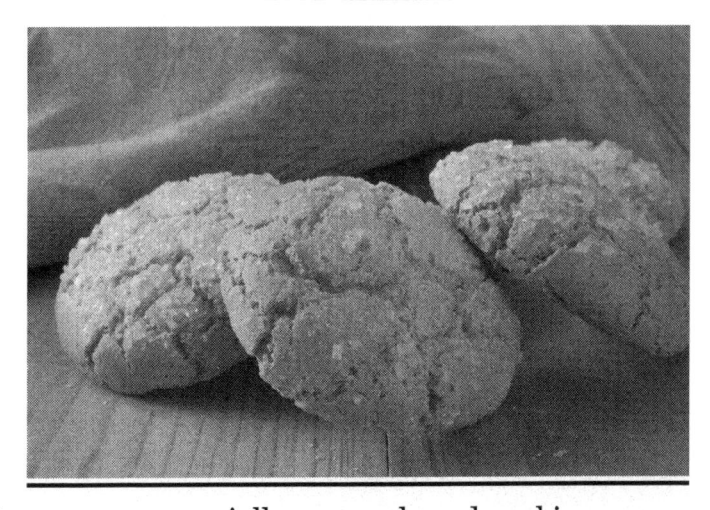

Because commercially pre-packaged cookies are filled with refined flours, and have a very high saturated fat content, they are definitely not a suitable tea or coffee time treat for those who prefer to feed their bodies with only the healthiest of foods. The cookies in this section are simple and easy to make. They don't have a long list of ingredients, and are packed with all the health benefits that come from fruits, raw nuts and seeds, and high fiber oats. These cookie recipes all have a base recipe that allows for all the different variations that follow, leaving no excuse to not whip up a much healthier, guilt-free, cookie option when the cookie monster is knocking on the door...

Ripe bananas and natural nut butter are the main ingredients of these recipes. Bananas are packed with potassium, fiber, vitamin C and B6. Potassium has been known to help keep the heart healthy and aid in muscle recover. The high fiber content of the banana helps regulate blood sugar levels. Along with the fiber rich oats, these cookies are a great pre- or post- workout snack. Their slow energy release properties also make them a great snack option to help keep you going through a long work day.

The natural nut butters provide you with heart healthy fats and another healthy energy boost. These cookie recipes don't contain any added sugar and rely on the fruit for their sweetness, making them a great treat for those who are controlling diabetes.

Date and Banana Cookies

The dates in these cookies add extra fiber, and dried fruit is known to be rich in iron, making these cookies a great recovery nibble after your morning run or cycle.

Serves: 12

Preheat the oven to 350 degrees (200 degrees Celsius). Give a non-stick baking sheet a light spraying of vegan friendly cooking spray, and set aside.

Ingredients:

- 2 Large Ripe Bananas, mashed
- 1 Cup (250ml) Organic raw oats
- 1 teaspoon (5ml) ground cinnamon
- 2 Tablespoons (30ml) Natural nut butter of your choice
- ¼ Cup (60ml) Chopped dates

Instructions:

1. In a mixing bowl combine the bananas, oats and cinnamon.
2. Once you have the mixture at a wet cookie dough consistency, add the chopped dates and mix thoroughly.

3. Scoop the dough onto the baking sheet, the size of each cookie is completely up to you, but since they will be very filling, they might be hard to finish if they are too big.
4. Bake for 15 minutes and allow to cool on the baking tray for 10 minutes before turning out onto a cooling rack.
5. It's best to store these in the refrigerator, once they have cooled completely.

Coconut, Cashew and Sultana Banana Cookies

The coconut flavor of these cookies compliments the cashew nut flavor, and the hint of cinnamon just brings it all together. The addition of sultanas, adds a golden touch along with an extra vitamin C boost. These cookies will go very well with a glass of organic pineapple juice to round off the tropical flavors.

Preheat the oven to 350degrees (200degrees Celsius). Give a non-stick baking sheet a light spraying of vegan friendly cooking spray, and set aside.

Serves: 12

Ingredients:

- 2 Large Ripe Bananas, mashed
- 1 Cup (250ml) Organic raw oats
- 1 teaspoon (5ml) ground cinnamon
- 2 Tablespoons (30ml) Natural nut butter of your choice
- ¼ Cup (60ml) Raw cashew nuts, chopped
- ¼ Cup (60ml) desiccated coconut
- ¼ Cup (60ml) Sultanas

Instructions:

1. In a mixing bowl combine the bananas, oats, desiccated coconut, chopped cashew nuts, and cinnamon.
2. Once you have the mixture at a wet cookie dough consistency, add the sultanas and mix thoroughly.
3. Scoop the dough onto the baking sheet, the size of each cookie is completely up to you, but since they will be very filling, they might be hard to finish if they are too big.
4. Bake for 15 minutes and allow to cool on the baking tray for 10 minutes before turning out onto a cooling rack.
5. It's best to store these in the refrigerator, once they have cooled completely.

Cranberry and Almond Banana Cookies

Dried cranberries are high in vitamin C and anti-oxidants, and the raw almonds add a punch of essential minerals such as manganese, magnesium, and a little extra potassium, as well as vitamin E, which is great for the skin.

Preheat the oven to 350degrees (200degrees Celsius). Give a non-stick baking sheet a light spraying of vegan friendly cooking spray, and set aside.

Serves: 12

Ingredients:

- 2 Large Ripe Bananas, mashed
- 1 Cup (250ml) Organic raw oats
- 1 teaspoon (5ml) ground cinnamon
- 2 Tablespoons (30ml) Natural nut butter of your choice
- ¼ Cup (60ml) Raw almonds, chopped
- ¼ Cup (60ml) Dried Cranberries

Instructions:

1. In a mixing bowl combine the bananas, oats,

chopped almonds, and cinnamon.
2. Once you have the mixture at a wet cookie dough consistency, add the cranberries and mix thoroughly.
3. Scoop the dough onto the baking sheet, the size of each cookie is completely up to you, but since they will be very filling, they might be hard to finish if they are too big.
4. Bake for 15 minutes and allow to cool on the baking tray for 10 minutes before turning out onto a cooling rack.
5. It's best to store these in the refrigerator, once they have cooled completely.

<u>Orange Ginger Banana Cookies</u>

This variation includes the high fiber content, phytonutrients and flavonoids of orange rind, along with its zesty flavor, that compliments the spiciness of the fresh ginger. The fresh ginger also brings along its anti-inflammatory properties.

Preheat the oven to 350degrees (200degrees Celsius). Give a non-stick baking sheet a light spraying of vegan friendly cooking spray, and set aside.

Serves: 12

Ingredients:

- 2 Large Ripe Bananas, mashed
- 1 Cup (250ml) Organic raw oats
- 1 teaspoon (5ml) ground cinnamon
- 2 Tablespoons (30ml) Natural nut butter of your choice
- ¼ Cup (60ml) Grated Orange zest
- 1 Tablespoon (15ml) Freshly grated ginger root.

Instructions:

1. In a mixing bowl combine the bananas, oats, grated ginger and cinnamon.
2. Once you have the mixture at a wet cookie dough

consistency, add the orange zest and mix thoroughly.
3. Scoop the dough onto the baking sheet, the size of each cookie is completely up to you, but since they will be very filling, they might be hard to finish if they are too big.
4. Bake for 15 minutes and allow to cool on the baking tray for 10 minutes before turning out onto a cooling rack.
5. It's best to store these in the refrigerator, once they have cooled completely.

Conclusion

Thank you for reading!

I hope that with so many vegan-friendly recipes you will be motivated and inspired to start your journey towards meaningful veganism, vibrant health and total wellbeing.

Remember, the beauty of incorporating nutritious vegan foods into your daily diet is that you are making simple, yet sustainable changes that will work for your wellness long-term. Not to mention your spiritual wellness and taking care of the environment.

If you enjoyed my book, it would be greatly appreciated if you left a review so others can receive the same benefits you have. Your review can help other people take this important step to take care of their health and inspire them to start a new chapter in their lives.

At the same time, <u>you can help me serve you and all my other readers</u> even more through my next vegan-friendly recipe books that I am committed to publishing on a regular basis.

I'd be thrilled to hear from you. I would love to know your favorite recipe(s).

Don't be shy, post a comment on Amazon!

Thank You for your time,

Love & Light,

Until next time-

Karen Vegan Greenvang

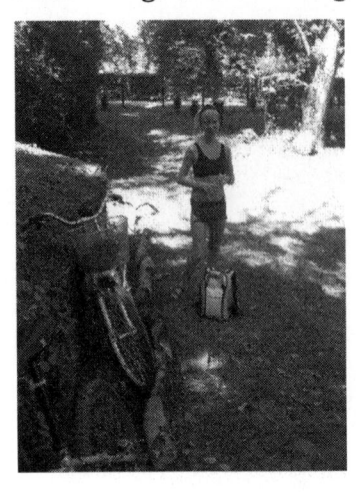

More Vegan Books by Karen

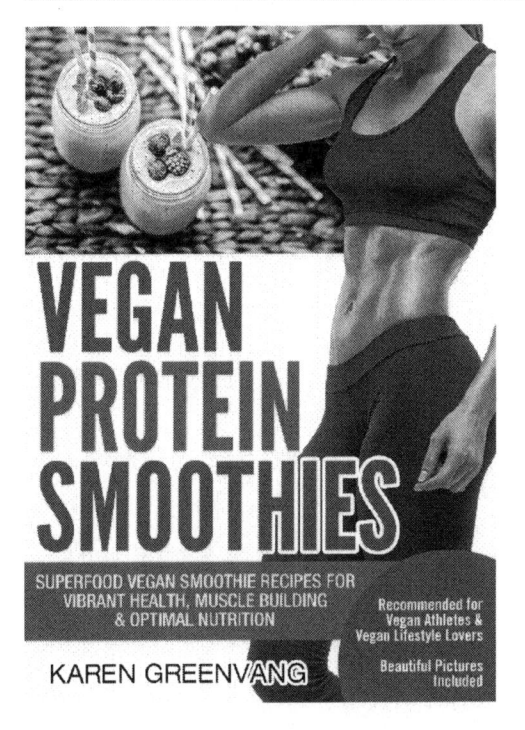

You will find more at:

www.amazon.com/author/karengreenvang

YOUR FREE GIFT

Smoothie Recipes

Insanely good + super healthy, 100% vegan smoothies with secret ingredients…YUM…

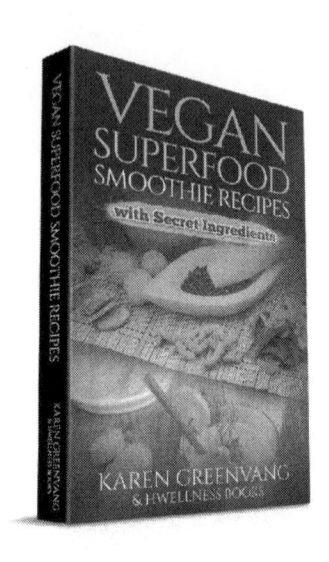

Visit:

www.bitly.com/karenfreegift

and secure your free copy now!

Printed in Poland
by Amazon Fulfillment
Poland Sp. z o.o., Wrocław